Python

for

Beginners

Python for Beginners: A practical guide for people who want to learn Python the right and easy way

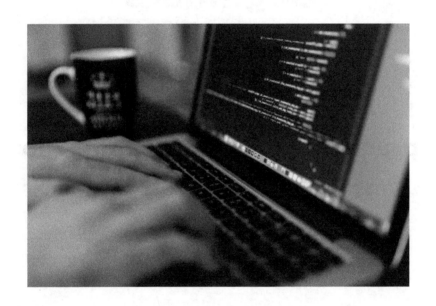

Table of Contents

The information in the following pages is broadly considered a truthful and accurate account of facts and as such, any inattention, use, or misuse of the information in question by the reader will render any resulting actions solely under their purview. There are no scenarios in which the publisher or the original author of this work can be in any fashion deemed liable for any hardship or damages that may befall them after undertaking information described herein.

Additionally, the information in the following pages is intended only for informational purposes and should thus be thought of as universal. As befitting its nature, it is presented without assurance regarding its prolonged validity or interim quality. Trademarks that are mentioned are done without written consent and can in no way be considered an endorsement from the trademark holder.

Introduction

Congratulations on purchasing *Python for Beginners* and thank you for doing so.

The following chapters will discuss everything that you need to know in order to get started with the Python coding language. There are a lot of different coding languages that you are able to work with, but none are going to give you the benefits, as well as ease of use, that you're going to find when you start with the Python coding language. This guidebook is going to spend some time looking at the steps that you need to take to get started with writing your very own codes, even if you are a beginner and have never done any coding in your life.

This guidebook is going to start out with some of the basics that come with the Python coding language. We will look at what the Python language is all about along with some of the benefits of using it, how to install this language, and some of the basic parts that come with your code. We will then move on to some of the different things you can do to get your feet wet with writing the codes that you want, including what the classes and objects are all about, how to work with the exceptions, and what those conditional statements are all about.

From there, we have so much more than we need to learn how to do with this kind of coding language, and this guidebook will make sure that you know how to make it happen. We will continue on looking at how to create lists and loops, the importance of Python files, how to do the functions in Python, data visualization, how to test your code, and where the regular expressions are able to come into the mix as well.

As you can see, there are a lot of different things that you are going to be able to do when you decide to work with the Python coding language. When you are ready to start learning how to do some of your own codes, and you want to be able to work on your own programs as soon as possible, make sure to check out this guidebook to help you get started.

There are plenty of books on this subject on the market, thanks again for choosing this one! Every effort was made to ensure it is full of as much useful information as possible. Please enjoy!

Chapter 1: Creating Inheritances in the Python Language

Working with some inheritances in your code can make a big difference in how things line up and work. In fact, these inheritances are going to be a good way to enhance any of the codes that you would like to work within Python. They are going to come into the code and save you a lot of time, while still ensuring that your code looks clean and nice along the way. Any programmer is able to do this by reusing a part of their previous code, without having to go through and rewrite the same code over and over again.

Basically, when you are ready to work with an inheritance in Python, it is time to take the original code, which is going to be known as the parent code here, and then change up parts of it before you reuse it in the derived or the child class. You are able to make any of the changes that you need to the child class to get it to work the way that you would like. Even as someone who is just starting with the Python process, you will be able to use the inheritances to help you rewrite different parts of your code over and over again.

During one of these inheritances, you are going to take the parent code, which is that original code, and copy it over into a new part of the program. This is then going to be the child code. With this child code, you can mess around with it and make it stronger or make other changes as you would wish. In some cases, you will want to copy it down as it is, and other times you may want to change up something inside of it to make the code work the way that you would like it to work.

To make a bit more sense out of some of the inheritances that you can do, and even out of how you can work with these inheritances, let's take a moment here to look at the code below to see exactly how these will work:

```
#Example of inheritance
#base class
class Student(object):
    def__init__(self, name, rollno):
    self.name = name
    self.rollno = rollno
#Graduate class inherits or derived from Student class
class GraduateStudent(Student):
```

```
        def__init__(self, name, rollno, graduate):
        Student__init__(self, name, rollno)
        self.graduate = graduate

def DisplayGraduateStudent(self):
        print"Student Name:", self.name)
        print("Student Rollno:", self.rollno)
        print("Study Group:", self.graduate)

#Post Graduate class inherits from Student class
class PostGraduate(Student):
        def__init__(self, name, rollno, postgrad):
        Student__init__(self, name, rollno)
        self.postgrad = postgrad

        def DisplayPostGraduateStudent(self):
        print("Student Name:", self.name)
        print("Student Rollno:", self.rollno)
        print("Study Group:", self.postgrad)

#instantiate from Graduate and PostGraduate classes
        objGradStudent = GraduateStudent("Mainu", 1,
"MS-Mathematics")
        objPostGradStudent = PostGraduate("Shainu",
2, "MS-CS")
```

objPostGradStudent.DisplayPostGraduateStudent()

When you type this into your interpreter, you are going to get the results:

('Student Name:', 'Mainu')
('Student Rollno:', 1)
('Student Group:', 'MSC-Mathematics')
('Student Name:', 'Shainu')
('Student Rollno:', 2)
('Student Group:', 'MSC-CS')

Overriding one of your base classes

Now that we have an example in code form above about what the inheritance is going to look like, now we need to take a look at what you would do when you want to take the base class and override it. There are going to be times when you have a new class, a child class, and you want to be able to override it a bit and change up some of the features in it to get it to work the way that you would like.

To make this happen, without making a mess along the way, you have to take a look at some of the things that are inside of the base class, and then determine how you can change those a bit to get that new child class. The child class is then going to work in order to use that new behavior to get the job done for you.

This may sound a bit scary to someone who is just getting started with the idea of inheritances and more, but it is really nice because you get a lot of freedom to pick out which parental features to keep around and which ones need to be avoided. This process, with the coding that we have above and more, is going to really help you to make all of the changes that you want with the child class, while still maintaining the parts that you do not want to change.

The number of times that you decide to do this is going to depend on the kind of code that you decide to work with. And you can make changes each time that you would like to make this happen. You can go through and have ten of these going down the line if you would like. And you can make it as simple or as complicated as you would like for your program. Putting it all together, and learning the basic steps to get all of this started is the trick that you need to ensure that you see the best results, and can add in as many of these layers as you would like.

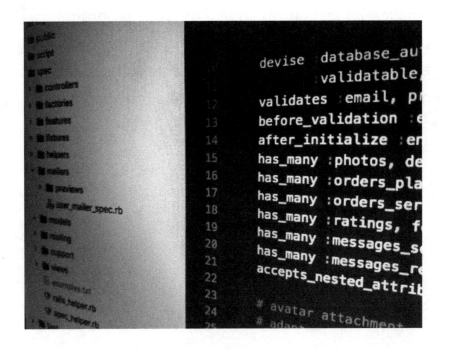

Chapter 2: Can I Create a Loop

Creating loops can be another great thing that you can work on when you have the Python language. These loops are going to make your life a whole lot easier, and often they can work well with the conditional statements that we talked about above in terms of making sure your code works the way that you want. Loops will speed up how long it takes to write your codes, can clean it all up, and can take hundreds of lines of code and wraps it up into just a few lines if you do it in the proper manner. Even as a beginner, you are able to make these loops work for you, so let's take a look at the way that you are able to make these works for your needs.

You will find that these loops are going to be so helpful any time that you are writing out a code where you would like to get a certain part of the program to go over and over the same lines, at least two times but often many, but you don't want to waste your time and make your code really messy by writing out the code each time. Let's say that you are going to try and write out a code for a multiplication chart to 100. Maybe you would write it all out line by line and waste a lot of time while making your code a mess. Or you could use a loop and write it out in just a few lines (we will show you how to do this in a little bit).

While this is something that can seem pretty complex, you will find that even as a beginner, it is really easy to work with these looks. The way that these kinds of code are going to work along with the compiler is that they are going to tell the compiler to just repeat the same part of the code over and over again. It is going to do this as many times as is needed, or until the condition that you added into the code ends up being met.

If you would like your code to have the ability to count up from one to ten, then you would simply need to tell the compiler that you want it to be able to stop once it gets to the number ten. We will look at a few of the examples that you can use to make all of this happen as we go through this guidebook.

Of course, when you are ready to start writing out these loops, you need to make sure that the conditions are set up the right way. if you don't set up your condition right from the beginning, then the program is going to end up with a mess because the code won't know when to stop, and it will keep going through the code an endless number of times, making you get stuck in a continuous loop. You have to put the condition put into the code, so it knows when you need it to stop and move on to the next part of the code.

When you work with what may be considered traditional methods of coding, or the ones that we talked about earlier on in this guidebook, your goal would be to write out all of the lines of code that you need. Even if there are some parts of the code that seem to be really similar, you would still need to go through and retype the same part of the code over and over again until it was done. But with loops, this is something that is no longer a concern.

Any time that you bring out the loops, you can dump the traditional way of doing coding out the window. You are able to combine many of the lines of code and make them work with just a few lines if you would like. The compiler will still be able to handle this and will know to repeat the lines as many times as you would like, as long as those conditions are all put in place.

With that introduction to the loops, it is time to look at the different types that you may work with when you start using the Python coding language. Some of the options include the for loop, the while loop, and the nested loop and we are going to take some time to go through each of these and see how each of them works and how they are going to improve your code writing.

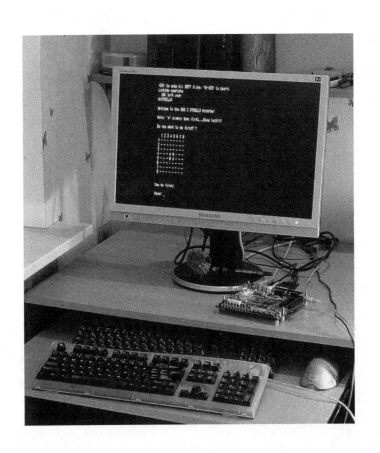

What is the while loop?

The first type of loop that you can work within your Python code is known as the while loop. The while loop is the type that you will use if you want to make sure that the code goes through a cycle a predetermined number of times. You can set this number of times when you write the code to make sure the loop goes for as long as you would like.

With the while loop, your goal is not to make the code go through its cycle an indefinite amount of times, but you do want to make sure that it goes through for a specific number of times. If you are counting from one to ten, you want to make sure it goes through the loop ten times to be right. With this option, the loop is going to go through at least one time and then check to see if the conditions are met or not. So, it will put up the number one, then check its conditions and put up the number two, and so on until it sees where it is.

To give us a little bit better of an understanding on how these loops work, let's take a look at some sample codes of the while loop and see what happens:

```
counter = 1
while(counter <= 3):
```

```
principal = int(input("Enter the principal
amount:"))
numberofyeras = int(input("Enter the number of
years:"))
rateofinterest = float(input("Enter the rate of
interest:"))
simpleinterest = principal * numberofyears *
rateofinterest/100
print("Simple interest = %.2f" %simpleinterest)
#increase the counter by 1
counter = counter + 1
print("You have calculated simple interest for 3
time!")
```

Before we move on, take this code and add it to your compiler and let it execute this code. You will see that when this is done, the output is going to come out in a way that the user can place any information that they want into the program. Then the program will do its computations and figure out the interest rates, as well as the final amounts, based on whatever numbers the user placed into the system.

With this particular example, we set the loop up to go through three times. This allows the user to put in results three times to the system before it moves on. You can always change this around though and add in more of the loops if it works the best for your program.

On to the for loop

Now that we have had a moment to take a look at the while loop, it is time to bring in the for loop and see how this one is going to be able to benefit us in a slightly different manner. The while loop that we just went through is going to have a lot of uses in your Python code. However, there may be times when it is not going to be able to handle all of the things that you want to do, and you may need to work with things in a different manner. And that is when we are going to start looking at them for a loop.

When we are ready for the for loop, you will be setting things up in your code so that the user isn't the one who will get in and give the information that is needed to tell the program to stop running the loop. Instead of having the user in charge, the for loop is going to set up in a way that it will go over the iteration in the order that you place the items in your statement, and then this information will show up in that exact manner. There isn't really a need for the user to input anything, at least until it gets to the end of the code.

A good example of how this is going to work inside your code so that you are able to make it work for your needs will include the following syntax:

```
# Measure some strings:
words = ['apple', 'mango', 'banana', 'orange']
for w in words:
print(w, len(w))
```

When you work with the for loop example that is above, you are able to add it to your compiler and see what happens when it gets executed. When you do this, the four fruits that come out on your screen will show up in the exact order that you have them written out. If you would like to have them show up in a different order, you can do that, but then you need to go back to your code and rewrite them in the right order, or your chosen order. Once you have then written out in the syntax and they are ready to be executed in the code, you can't make any changes to them.

And finally, the nested loop

And then there is one final loop type that we are going to need to work within our Python code is the nested loop. You will find that the nested loop can use some of the parts that we have talked about with the for loop and the while loop but in a slightly different manner. When you are bringing out the nested loop, you will basically take one loop and then have it placed right inside of another loop. Then both of the loops will continue on their path until they are both able to finish.

This may seem like it is really complicated to get started with, and you may be wondering at this time when you would actually need to use this kind of loop, but you may find that as you get to writing some of your own codes, there are actually quite a few times when this does come in handy. For example, you may have a time when you need to write out a multiplication table inside the code, giving you answers from one times one, all the way up to ten times ten.

Imagine how long this would take to go through and write out each line of code. You would need to write out one time one, one times two, one times three, one times four and so on until you got yourself all the way up to ten times ten. This is a lot of lines of code and can take you forever. But with a nested loop, you are able to get this to work for you, without having to write out so much code at once. A good syntax of how you can write out the multiplication table idea that we talked about before will include

#write a multiplication table from 1 to 10
For x in xrange(1, 11):
*   For y in xrange(1, 11):*
*   Print '%d = %d' % (x, y, x*x)*

When you got the output of this program, it is going to look similar to this:

1*1 = 1

1*2 = 2

1*3 = 3

1*4 = 4

All the way up to 1*10 = 2

Then it would move on to do the table by twos such as this:

2*1 =2

2*2 = 4

And so, on until you end up with 10*10 = 100 as your final spot in the sequence.

Go ahead and put this into the compiler and see what happens. You will simply have four lines of code, and end up with a whole multiplication table that shows up on your program. Think of how many lines of code you would have to write out to get this table the traditional way that you did before? This table only took a few lines to accomplish, which shows how powerful and great the nested loop can be.

The loops are great options to add into your code. There are a lot of reasons when you would need to take a loop and add it inside your code. You will be able to use it as a way to get a lot of coding done in just a few lines, and a way to clean up the code so that you can still get the same thing done without writing out too much. The compiler is set up to keep reading through the loop until the condition that you set is no longer valid. This can open up a lot of things that you are able to do with your code, while also keeping things clean and manageable all at the same time.

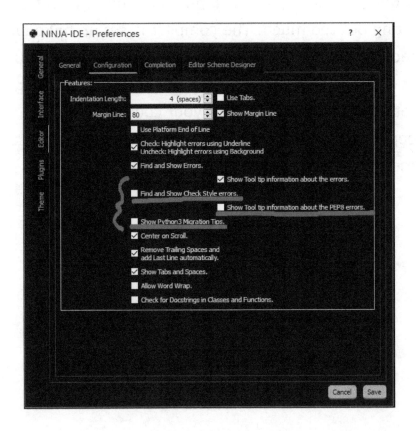

NINJA-IDE - Preferences   ?   ✕

General | Configuration | Completion | Editor Scheme Designer

Features:

Indentation Length: 4 (spaces) ⏶⏷   ☐ Use Tabs.

Margin Line: 80   ⏶⏷   ☑ Show Margin Line

☐ Use Platform End of Line

☑ Check: Highlight errors using Underline
   Uncheck: Highlight errors using Background

☑ Find and Show Errors.

☑ Show Tool tip information about the errors.

☐ Find and Show Check Style errors.

☐ Show Tool tip information about the PEP8 errors.

☐ Show Python3 Migration Tips.

☑ Center on Scroll.

☑ Remove Trailing Spaces and
   add Last Line automatically.

☑ Show Tabs and Spaces.

☐ Allow Word Wrap.

☐ Check for Docstrings in Classes and Functions.

Cancel   Save

Chapter 3: Working with the Python Files

The next thing that we need to focus on when it comes to working with Python is making sure we know how to do with these kinds of codes is working with the Python files. There are going to be times when you are working with some data in these codes, and you will want to store it then while ensuring that it is accessible for you to pull up and use when the data is needed later. You do have some choices in the way that you save this data, how it is going to be found later on, and how it is going to react in your code.

When you work with the files, you will find that the data is going to be saved on a disk, or you are able to re-use in the code over and over again as much as you would like. This chapter is going to help us learn a bit more about how to handle some of the work that we need to do to ensure the files behave the way that they should, and so much more.

Now, we are going to enter into file mode on the Python language, and this allows you to do a few different options along the way. A good way to think about this is that you can think about it like working on a file in Word. At some point, you may try to save one of the documents that you are working with so that it doesn't get lost and you are able to find them later on. These kinds of files in Python are going to be similar. But you won't be saving pages as you did on Word, you are going to save parts of your code.

You will find with this one that there are a few operations or methods that you are able to choose when it comes to working with files. And some of these options will include:

1. Closing up a file you are working on.
2. Creating a brand new file to work on.
3. Seeking out or moving a file that you have over to a new location to make it easier to find.
4. Writing out a new part of the code on a file that was created earlier.

Creating your new files

The first task that we are going to look at doing here is working on creating a file. It is hard to do much of the other tasks if we don't first have a file in place to help us out. if you would like to be able to make a new file and then add in some code into it, you first need to make sure the file is opened up inside of your IDLE. Then you can choose the mode that you would like to use when you write out your code.

When it comes to creating files on Python, you will find there are three modes that you are able to work with. The three main modes that we are going to focus on here includes append (a), mode(x) and write(w).

Any time that you would like to open up a file and make some changes in it, then you would want to use the write mode. This is the easiest out of the three to work with. The write method is going to make it easier for you to get the right parts of the code set up and working for you in the end.

The write function is going to be easy to use and will ensure that you are able to make any and all additions and changes that you would like to the file. You can add in the new information that you would like to the file, change what is there, and so much more. If you would like to see what you are able to do with this part of the code with the write method, then you will want to open up your compiler and do the following code:

```
#file handling operations
#writing to a new file hello.txt
f = open('hello.txt', 'w', encoding = 'utf-8')
f.write("Hello Python Developers!")
f.write("Welcome to Python World")
f.flush()
f.close()
```

From here, we need to discuss what you are able to do with the directories that we are working with. The default directory is always going to be the current directory. You are able to go through and switch up the directory where the code information is stored, but you have to take the time, in the beginning, to change that information up, or it isn't going to end up in the directory that you would like.

Whatever directory you spent your time in when working on the code is the one you need to make your way back to when you want to find the file later on. If you would like it to show up in a different directory, make sure that you move over to that one before you save it and the code. With the option that we wrote above, when you go to the current directory (or the directory that you chose for this endeavor, then you will be able to open up the file and see the message that you wrote out there.

For this one, we wrote a simple part of the code. You, of course, will be writing out codes that are much more complicated as we go along. And with those codes, there are going to be times when you would like to edit or overwrite some of what is in that file. This is possible to do with Python, and it just needs a small change to the syntax that you are writing out. A good example of what you are able to do with this one incudes:

```
#file handling operations
#writing to a new file hello.txt
f = open('hello.txt', 'w', encoding = 'utf-8')
f.write("Hello Python Developers!")
```

```
f.write("Welcome to Python World")
mylist = ["Apple", "Orange", "Banana"]
#writelines() is used to write multiple lines in to the
file
f.write(mylist)
f.flush()
f.close()
```

The example above is a good one to use when you want to make a few changes to a file that you worked on before because you just need to add in one new line. This example wouldn't need to use that third line because it just has some simple words, but you can add in anything that you want to the program, just use the syntax above and change it up for what you need.

What are the binary files?

One other thing that we need to focus on for a moment before moving on is the idea of writing out some of your files and your data in the code as a binary file. This may sound a bit confusing, but it is a simple thing that Python will allow you to do. All that you need to do to make this happen is to take the data that you have and change it over to a sound or image file, rather than having it as a text file.

With Python, you are able to change any of the code that you want into a binary file. It doesn't matter what kind of file it was in the past. But you do need to make sure that you work on the data in the right way to ensure that it is easier to expose in the way that you want later on. The syntax that is going to be needed to ensure that this will work well for you will be below:

```
# write binary data to a file
# writing the file hello.dat write binary mode
F = open('hello.dat', 'wb')
# writing as byte strings
f.write(b"I am writing data in binary file!/n")
f.write(b"Let's write another list/n")
f.close()
```

If you take the time to use this code in your files, it is going to help you to make the binary file that you would like. Some programmers find that they like using this method because it helps them to really get things in order and will make it easier to pull the information up when you need it.

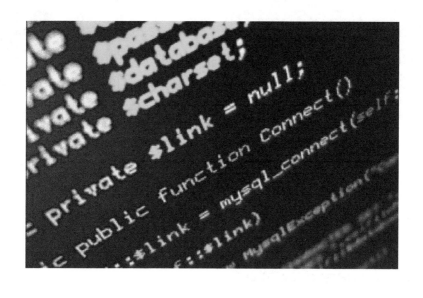

Opening your file up

So far, we have worked with writing a new file and getting it saved, and working with a binary file as well. In these examples, we got some of the basics of working with files down so that you are able to make them work for you and you can pull them up any time that you would like.

Now that this part is done, it is time to learn how to open up the file and use it, and later even make changes to it, any time that you would like. Once you open that file up, it is going to be so much easier to use it again and again as much as you would like. When you are ready to see the steps that are needed in order to open up a file and use it, you will need the following syntax.

```
# read binary data to a file
#writing the file hello.dat write append binary mode

with open("hello.dat", 'rb') as f:
    data = f.read()
    text = data.decode('utf-8'(
print(text)
```

the output that you would get form putting this into the system would be like the following:

Hello, world!
This is a demo using with
This file contains three lines
Hello world
This is a demo using with

This file contains three lines.

Seeking out a file you need

And finally, we need to take a look at how you are able to seek out some of the files that you need on this kind of coding language. We already looked at how to make the files, how to store them in different manners, how to open them and rewrite on them, and then how to seek the file. But there are times where you are able to move one of the files that you have over to a new location.

For example, if you are working on a file and as you do that, you find that things are not showing up the way that you would like it to, then it is time to fix this up. Maybe you didn't spell the time of the identifier the right way, or the directory is not where you want it to be, then the seek option may be the best way to actually find this lost file and then make the changes, so it is easier to find later on.

With this method, you are going to be able to change up where you place the file, to ensure that it is going to be in the right spot all of the time or even to make it a bit easier for you to find it when you need. You just need to use a syntax like what is above in order to help you make these changes.

Working through all of the different methods that we have talked about in this chapter are going to help you to do a lot of different things inside of your code. Whether you would like to make a new file, you want to change up the code, move the file around, and more; you will be able to do it all using the codes that we have gone through in this chapter.

```python
def add5(x):
    return x+5

def dotwrite(ast):
    nodename = getNodename()
    label=symbol.sym_name.get(int(ast[0]),ast[0])
    print '    %s [label="%s' % (nodename,label),
    if isinstance(ast[1], str):
        if ast[1].strip():
            print '= %s"];' % ast[1]
        else:
            print '"]'
    else:
        print '"];'
        children = []
        for n, child in enumerate(ast[1:]):
            children.append(dotwrite(child))
        print '    %s -> {' % nodename,
        for name in children:
            print '%s' % name,
```

Chapter 4 The Importance of the Python Functions

Another important topic that you are able to work with in order to see some great results with your codes are going to be the Python functions. These functions are going to be known as a set of expressions, or statements, that will either have a name, or you can choose to keep them a bit anonymous. They are going to be the first types of class objects that you will be able to find inside the code, so you won't have to worry as much about the restrictions or how these functions are going to be allowed to work.

When you decide to pull up these functions or create a new one, you will find that they are pretty similar to other kinds of values that you are using in the code. You will be able to use them like the strings or the numbers that we have talked about before, and you can add-in attributes that help with these, as like as you use the prefix of "dir."

There are a lot of different types of functions that you are able to deal with, and you can even choose from a good variety of attributes when it is time to create, and then later bring up, the functions that you want to use in your code. Some of the different choices that are available to help you with this will include the following:

- __doc__: This is going to return the docstring of the function that you are requesting.
- Func_default: This one is going to return a tuple of the values of your default argument.
- Func_globals: This one will return a reference that points to the dictionary holding the global variables for that function.
- Func_dict: This one is responsible for returning the namespace that will support the attributes for all your arbitrary functions.
- Func_closure: This will return to you a tuple of all the cells that hold the bindings for the free variables inside of the function.

As you can see, working with these functions is not something that has to be extraordinarily hard to work with. It takes some time to add them in, but if you use some of the identifiers that are above, you will be just fine getting this all done.

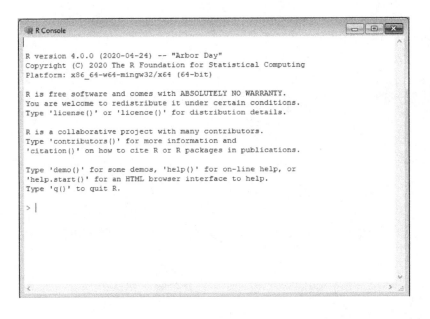

Chapter 5: Bringing in Some Data Visualization

Another part that we need to take a look at with the Python language is the idea of data visualization. This is a big part of the job of a data scientist. In the early stages of the project, it is likely that you are going to spend a lot of time doing what is known as EDA, or Exploratory Data Analysis, in order to gain a bit more insight into your data.

Being able to create some visualizations can really help make things easier and for you to understand, especially when it comes to data sets that are larger and are seen as higher dimensional. When you are getting close to done with your project, it is also important for you to be able to present these results in a manner that is compelling, concise, and clear so that an audience, even if they are not technically inclined, are able to understand the information as well.

Before we get too far into all of this, you may want to make sure that you have the Python library known as Matplotlib on your system. You will be able to use this to make some of the things that you will do with data visualization a bit easier. However, you may find that setting up the figures, parameters, data, and plotting all of this is going to be tedious and a bit messy if you have to go through and redo them each time you start a new project.

In this chapter, we are going to explore a few different types of data visualizations you can work with, along with some of the easy and fast functions that you can do with each of these thanks to the Matplotlib that you can get form Python. Make sure to get this library on your system, if it is not there already, to help you get this done.

Scatter Plots

The first thing that you can look at with data visualization is the scatter plots. These are going to be great when it is time to show the relationship between two different variables since you can look at them and see the raw distribution of any kind of data that you have. You can also view this relationship for different groups of data if they are split up, simply by changing the color of each ground.

Let's say that you want to take a look at the relationship that is present between three different variables. This is pretty easy to do. You just need to use the parameters to change the colors of each one so that you can split them all up into the groups that you want. Then, thanks to the colors telling us which dots are for each parameter, we are better able to see the relationship that is going to show up here.

So that brings up the question of how you are able to do this with Python. We first need to import the pyplot from Matplotlib. It is going to have the alias of plt. To create a new plot figure, we are going to call up "plt.subplots(). We pass the x-axis and the y-axis data over to the function, and then these are going to be passed over to the ax.scatter() to plot the scatter plot. We can also go through and set up the alpha transparency, the point color, and the point size. You are even able to go through and set up the y-axis so that it comes in with a logarithmic scale. The title and the axis labels are then going to be set in a specific manner that you want.

To see the code that you will want to use to make this happen and to create your own scatter plot (importing the information that you want it to look over), you just need to work with the code that is found below:

import
matplotlib.pyplot
as plt
     import numpy as np

```python
def scatterplot(x_data, y_data,
x_label="", y_label="", title="",
color = "r", yscale_log=False):

    # Create the plot object
    _, ax = plt.subplots()

    # Plot the data, set the size (s),
    color and transparency (alpha)
    # of the points
    ax.scatter(x_data, y_data, s =
    10, color = color, alpha = 0.75)
```

Line Plots

The next thing that we are going to take a look at when we are working with Python and data visualization is going to be the line plots. These are going to be the best thing to use when you are able to clearly see that one variable is going to be quite a bit different than the other. This also means they have a high amount of co-variance.

There may be times when you have a lot of different items that you need to work with at the same time. and maybe they touch and meet up at the same points on a regular basis. If you tried to do a scatter plot of all of this information, it would get messy and be hard to look through and analyze at all. The lines, usually in different colors, can still give you an idea of where each type is going, how they can be separated out, and more.

If you would like to be able to make your own line plot with the help of the Python code, then you can use the following code to help you get all of this done:

def lineplot(x_data,
y_data, x_label="",
y_label="", title=""):

```python
# Create the plot object
_, ax = plt.subplots()
# Plot the best fit line, set
the linewidth (lw), color and
# transparency (alpha) of
the line
ax.plot(x_data, y_data, lw =
2, color = '#539caf', alpha =
1)
# Label the axes and provide
a title
ax.set_title(title)
ax.set_xlabel(x_label)
```

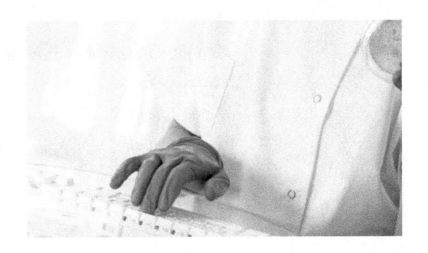

Histograms

Another type of data visualization tool that you are able to work with when you are ready to get some great ways to look through your data is going to be the histogram. You will find that these histograms are going to be useful when you are viewing, or when you want to discover, how the data points you are working with are being distributed.

When you are looking at some of these histograms, you may notice that it is going to show you that there is going to be a nice concentration of points that shows up right in the middle, and this is going to be the median that you need to focus on. You will also see that many of these are going to be able to follow what is known as a Gaussian distribution.

When you use the bars that are found in a histogram, rather than the scatter points or even the lines on this one, you are going to really be able to visualize of the relative difference between the frequency of each part. The use of the bins is going to be helpful here because it ensures that you are able to really come in and see the bigger picture. But if there weren't these kinds of bins in place, there would end up being a ton of noise in the visualization, which would make it harder to look through the data and see what is going on there.

We will look at the code that you can use in Matplotlib in order to create one of these histograms. Before we do that, though, there are going to be a few parameters that are important, and we need to take a look at them. The first of these is going to be the n_bins parameter. This is important because it is able to control how many of the discrete bins you want to allow with this histogram.

If you are working with more of these bins, it is going to give you finer information, but it is possible that having too many of these will introduce a lot of noise and can take you away from the bigger picture that you want to have. Then there is the issue with having not enough bins. This is going to give you more of a bird's eye view. It shows you the bigger picture of what might be seen in the data, but without the finer details that you may need.

The second parameter that you need to look at is going to be the cumulative parameter. This is a Boolean one that will allow you to select whether the histogram is considered cumulative or not. This is basically where you are going to pick out the CDF, or the Cumulative Density Function, or the PDF, or the Probability Density Function.

Now we can get to the code. The code that you can use with the Python program to make your own histogram is going to include:

```
def histogram(data, n_bins, cumulative=False,
x_label = "", y_label = "", title = ""):
_, ax = plt.subplots()
```

```
ax.hist(data, n_bins = n_bins, cumulative =
cumulative, color = '#539caf')
ax.set_ylabel(y_label)
ax.set_xlabel(x_label)
ax.set_title(title)
```

Now, you may find that there are going to be times
when you could bring out the histogram in order to
compare how the distribution of the two variables are
going to work with the data. You may assume that
you have to go through and create two different
histograms and look at this information all on its own
or compare side to side. But there is actually a way
that you are able to do in order to help you out. You
can overlay the histograms with varying
transparencies to see where they match together and
where not.

There are a lot of times when you will want to work with this kind of histogram, but first, you need to make sure that there are a few things set up in the code to do this. First, we need to be able to set up a horizontal range in order to help you deal with both of the distributions. According to the number of bins you want to use and this range, you can then compute the width that you need for each bin. And then you need to work on plotting both of these histograms on the same plot, allowing one of them to show up a bit more transparent than the other so you can compare. The code that you need to make this one happen includes the following:

```
# Overlay 2 histograms to compare them
def overlaid_histogram(data1, data2, n_bins = 0,
data1_name="", data1_color="#539caf",
data2_name="", data2_color="#7663b0",
x_label="", y_label="", title=""):
# Set the bounds for the bins so that the two
distributions are fairly compared
max_nbins = 10
data_range = [min(min(data1), min(data2)),
max(max(data1), max(data2))]
```

```
binwidth = (data_range[1] - data_range[0]) /
max_nbins

if n_bins == 0
bins = np.arange(data_range[0], data_range[1] +
binwidth, binwidth)
else:
```

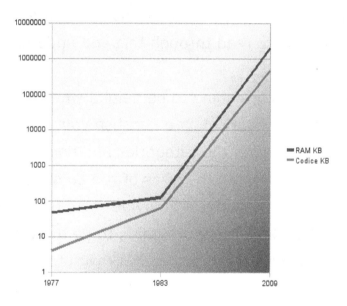

Bar Plots

You can also work with bar plots when it comes to working in the Python language. You will find that working on these bar plots can be effective when you are working on visualizing some data that is categorical and has only a few categories, usually less than ten. If you end up with too many categories here, then the bars are going to look cluttered, and it is hard for you to read through this and understand it.

These bar plots are going to be helpful when you want to work with categorical data because you will then be able to look through the categories and find out the comparisons based on the sizes of the bars. You can even take the categories and divide them up based on their color as well. There are going to be three main types of bar plots that you can work with to sort out your data, including stacked, grouped, and regular.

The regular bar plot is the first one that we will be able to look at. In the barplot() function, the x_data is going to represent the tickers on the x-axis, and the y_data is going to be the height of the bar as it goes up the y-axis. The error bar is going to be the extra line centered on each bar that you will be able to draw out and show what the standard deviation is.

Then there is the grouped bar plot. This one is going to be important at times because it helps us to compare more than one variable. The first variable that we are going to go through and compare is going to be the scores that are in each group, using G1, G2, and more. We are also comparing the genders themselves, but we are going to color code them.

When we look at the code in a bit, the y_data_list variable is not actually going to be a list of lists, and you will notice that each sublist that we have is going to be able to show us another group. We can then go through and loop through each group, and then each of these groups is going to have us draw the bar for each tock on the x-axis. These groups are going to be color-coded for us.

And then the third type of bar plot is going to be the stacked bar plot. These are going to be great when it is time to visualize the categorical make-up of the different variables. Om the stacked bar plot we are going to be able to color code it and do more in order to figure out what seemed to work the best on each day or in each category for us.

The codes that are needed to work with the bar plots and to make sure that they work well for your needs will include the following:

```python
def barplot(x_data,
y_data, error_data,
x_label="",
y_label="", title=""):
    _, ax = plt.subplots()
    # Draw bars, position them in
    the center of the tick mark on
    the x-axis
    ax.bar(x_data, y_data, color =
    '#539caf', align = 'center')
    # Draw error bars to show
    standard deviation, set ls to
    'none'
    # to remove line between
    points
    ax.errorbar(x_data, y_data,
    yerr = error_data, color =
    '#297083', ls = 'none', lw = 2,
    capthick = 2)
    ax.set_ylabel(y_label)
    ax.set_xlabel(x_label)
    ax.set_title(title)
```

```
513  class Set {
514    private Object elements[];
515    private int MAX = 500;
516    private int pos;
517
518    public Set() {
519      elements = new Object[MAX];
520    }
521    public void reset() {
522      for (int i = 0; i < MAX; i++) {
523        elements[i] = null;
524      }
525    }
526    public boolean addElement(Object x) {
527      if (containsElement(x))
528        return false;
529      int i;
530      i = 0;
531      while (i < MAX) {
532        if (elements[i] == null) {
533          elements[i] = x;
534          return true;
535        }
536        i++;
537      }
538      return false;
539    }
540    public boolean containsElement(Object x) {
541      int i;
542      i = 0;
543      while (i < MAX) {
544        if (elements[i] != null
545            && elements[i].equals(x)) {
546          return true;
547        }
548        i++;
549      }
550      return false;
551    }
552    public Object findElement(Object x) {
553      for (int i = 0; i < MAX; i++) {
554        if (elements[i] != null
555            && elements[i].equals(x)) {
```

74

Box Plots

We already took some time to look at histograms earlier in this chapter. Histograms are a great way for you to visualize the distribution of variables. But there are going to be some times when you will want to work with some more information than that. Perhaps you would like to be able to find a clearer view of the standard deviation. You may sometimes find the information for the median is going to be quite a bit different from the mean, and it results in a lot of outliers that you need to figure out as well. What if there is such a skew in it and a lot of the values are going to be concentrated to one side.

This is where you will be able to use the boxplots to your advantage. Box plots are going to give it all of the information that you need even if there are a lot of changes that go on in the data. The bottom and the top of these solid lined boxes are going to be the first and the third quartiles, and then the band inside the box is always going to be our median or the second quartile. The whiskers or the dashed lines with bars on the end, are going to extend from the box to show you what range of the data.

Since the box plot that we want to work with is going to be drawn for each group or variable, it is going to be easy to set up. The x_data is going to be a list of the groups and variables. The Matplotlib function of boxplot() is going to help us make a plot for each of the columns of the y_data or each vector in the sequence y_data. This means that each value that shows up in the x_data is going to correspond to a volume or vector that is in the y_data. All we have to do for this is to set them up to look right in the plot.

Now that we have talked a bit about how the box plot looks like, it is time to take a look at the code that you need to use in order to make all of this happen. The best code to make your own box plot includes

```
def boxplot(x_data, y_data, base_color="#539caf",
median_color="#297083", x_label="", y_label="",
title=""):
    _, ax = plt.subplots()
    # Draw boxplots, specifying desired style
    ax.boxplot(y_data
    # patch_artist must be True to control box fill
    , patch_artist = True
    # Properties of median line
```

, medianprops = {'color': median_color}

 # Properties of box

, boxprops = {'color': base_color, 'facecolor': base_color}

These are the five things that you can do when it comes to doing data visualization in your work. Abstracting things into functions can always make it easier for you to read your code and use it. And you can use the simple codes that we have in this chapter to help you make some of your own codes and see some amazing results in the process.

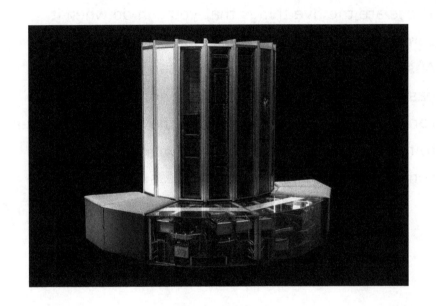

Chapter 6: Testing Your Code

When you are working with the Python language, there is some time when you would want to test out the codes that you are working with. Getting used to writing out some of your own testing code, and then running it at the same time that you do with the rest of your code is seen as a good habit in coding, and learning how to do it the right way is going to make sure that you get things to work the way that you want. When you use this kind of method in the proper manner, it is going to make it easier to define your code and get it to work well.

Before we get started, it is important to take a look at a few of the rules that are there for testing to keep things organized. These rules include

1. A testing unit has to focus on just one tiny part of the functionality of your code, and then it needs to prove that this is correct, rather than taking on a really large part.
2. Each test unit needs to be fully independent and on its own. This means that each test that you need to run should be able to run on its own, while also being in the test suite, regardless of

the order it is called up. The implication of this kind of rule is that each test has to be loaded up with a fresh set of data and then it needs to be able to do the cleanup to make this happen. This is usually going to be handled by the methods of setup() and teardown().

3. You should make it a goal to get tests that are able to run fast. If you find that one of your individual's tests ends up needing more than a few milliseconds to run, this is going to slow down your development, or these tests may not run as often as you desire.

    a. In some cases, the tests aren't going to be fast because they need to work on some complex data structure. And then you need to load up this data each time the tests run. If you have to do some of these heavier tasks in your tests, then you need to make sure that they are kept in a separate test suite that is run by some scheduled task, and then run all of the other tests as often as they are needed in all of this.

4. Learn about all of your tools and learn how to run a single test or a test case. Then, when you are developing a function inside of a module,

run this function's tests frequently, ideally automatically when you try to save some part of the code.

5. Always make it so that the full test suite is going to run before the coding session, and then have it run again when the coding is done. This is going to ensure that there is some confidence that nothing will break in the rest of the code and that the cleanup is going to work the way that you want.

6. It is always a good idea to implement a hook that runs all tests before you try to push code to a shared repository.

7. If you are already in the middle of one of your sessions of development and you have to stop, it is still a good idea to go through and write out a broken test about what you would like to have done next. When you come back to the coding later than, this is going to give you a pointer about where you were at that time and can ensure that you are going to be able to get back on track a bit faster.

8. The first thing that should be looked at when you want to debug your code is to write out a new test that pinpoints that bug. While this is not always going to be an easy thing to do,

those bug catching tests are going to help you out so much and are one of the most valuable things that you are able to do to keep your code working well.

9. Try to use long and descriptive names for testing functions. The style guide here is going to be a bit different compared to what you are going to do when you run your code, where you will most often want to stay with some shorter names. The reason for this is that testing the functions are never going to be called up explicitly. Square() and sqr() are ok when you are running the code, but they are not going to be used when you are running a test.

10. When you see that there is something going wrong, or there is something that should be changed, and if your code already has a good set of tests, you or the other maintainers are going to need to work on your testing suite in order to make the modifications or to fix some of the problems. Therefore, this means that you will need to test the code to be read more than the rest. A unit test whose purpose is unclear is not going to help you out with this much.

11. Another way that you are able to use your testing code is a type of introduction to a lot of

new developers. When you need to work on the code base, running and reading the related testing code is a great way to help them to start. You will then be able to discover some of the hot pots, where a lot of difficulties can arise. They will be able to add in some functionality and learn a lot more about your code in the process.

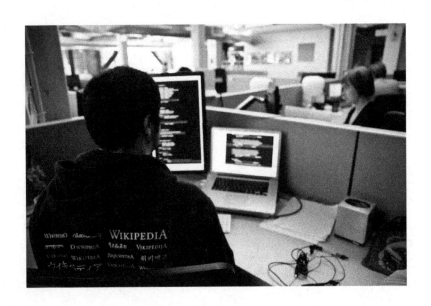

Decisions to make before testing

Before you dive into writing your own tests in Python, you want to make up a few decisions as well. You need to figure out what you would like to test and figure out whether you are working with an integration test or a unit test. When you have this figured out, you will then need to structure out the test and how it is loosely going to follow with the workflow. You need it to create the inputs, then you need to move on to the code being tested and capturing your output. And in the end, you need to compare the output with the results that you were expecting to get.

For this kind of application, you may want to test out the sum() method. There are a lot of different things that this kind of method is able to check including:

1. Can it sum a list of whole numbers or integers?
2. Can it sum a tuple or a set?
3. Can it sum a list of floats?
4. What happens when you put in a bad value, such as a single integer or a whole string?
5. What is going to happen when one of the values ends up being negative?

Manual vs. Automated Testing

The good news to consider here is that when writing out some of the codes that you want to work with, it is likely that you have been able to test without realizing it. Remember when you ran the application and used it for the first time? Did you check through the features and experiment using them? This is something that is known as exploratory testing and is a form of manual testing.

Exploratory testing is going to be a form of testing that any coder is able to do without a plan in place. When you are in this kind of testing, you are just going through and exploring the application and all that it is able to do.

To have a complete set of manual tests, all you need to do is make a list of all the features of your application, the different types of input it can accept, and the results that you are expecting. Now, every time you try to make a change to your code, you will need to go through every item that you have added to that list and check it all out.

Of course, this isn't something that sounds like that much fun. You don't really want to go through all of that and try to create some of the code each time. This is where automated testing is going to be able to come in. automated testing is going to be the execution of your test plan (which is the parts of your application that you would like to test, in the order that you wish to test them, and then the responses that you plan to get), but a script rather than the person going through and doing it. Python already has several libraries and tools that you are able to create automated tests for the application.

Integration Tests and Unit Tests

The world of testing is going to come with a lot of terminologies, and now that you know the difference between manual and automated testing. Now it is time to go a little bit deeper. Think of how you might test the lights that are on your car. You would first turn on the lights, which is your test step. And then you would go out of the car or ask a friend to check whether the lights turned on. This is going to be known as the test assertion. Testing more than one component here is going to be known as integration testing.

Think about all of the things that you would like to have worked correctly just to get a simple task the right results that you are looking for. These components are like the parts that come with your application, all of the modules, the functions, and the classes.

A big challenge that comes with this kind of testing is going to show up when the test doesn't give you the results that you would like. It can be hard for you to figure out what the issue is if you are not able to isolate the part of the system that isn't doing the work that you want. If the lights don't turn on in the car, what could be the problem? Is it the battery dying, the bulbs being broken, the computer of the car failing or something else?

If you have a newer car, it is possible that it is going to be able to tell you what is going on. And it is able to do this with the help of a unit test. The unit test is going to be a smaller test, one that is able to check that a single component is operating in the way that it should. It is the best way to isolate what is broken in the application, and then you can go right there and get it fixed.

Both the integration test and the unit test are things that you are able to work on inside of Python. To be able to write this kind of unit test to check out the built-in function sum(), you would need to check out the output of sum() against the output that you know needs to come out.

As you can see, there are a lot of different reasons why you will want to work with testing in Python. It will ensure that you are able to get the best results with your work, and can make it easier to debug the system and get it to work the way that you would like. Check out some of the things that we just talked about in this guidebook and this chapter, and see how easy it can be to test out some of your codes.

Chapter 7: What are the Regular Expressions in This Coding Language

Regular expressions are another fun thing that you will get to enjoy when it is time to work on the Python coding language. When you first get started with this language, take some time to see what is found in the library. You may be amazed at all that is there inside of it. This library is going to have a lot of regular expressions, ones that are going to help you do the searches that are needed to make your code work behind the scenes

These expressions are something that you will use in your coding because it will filter out all of the different kinds of texts that you have. it is possible to check and then see whether a string or some other text is going to be present in your code, and then see if it matches back up to the regular expression as well. And when you work with these kinds of expressions, you will find that the syntax is going to be the same each time, which makes it a bit easier to keep track of and remember. Learning how to do this on Python, and you will find that you can use it with some other coding languages as well.

Now that we have taken a look at these regular expressions a bit, you may need a definition to go with them so that you ensure they are used properly when it is time to bring them out. a good place to start with this is to open up your text editor, and then see if you are able to locate a word that has been spelled in two different ways in the same code. We will look through some of the steps to take to make this happen and to ensure that all of the confusion that comes with regular expressions so that you can handle this and any other problems that may come up when you are working with regular expressions.

You will find that working with regular expressions can be a lot of fun because they will open up a world of things that you are now able to do with your code. This is why it is so important for you to learn the right way for you to use them. Any time that you are ready to start adding these to your code, the first thing to do is import the expression library. You are able to use this when the program is first started up because it is something that you will use often.

As you work on your codes in Python, you will notice that regular expressions are going to start showing up on a regular basis. And if you are able to learn how to make these works, you will then be able to see some new things happen in your code as well. Now that we know a bit more about these regular expressions, let's take it a bit further and figure out how to use these to get the results that we are looking for.

The basic patterns to look for

There are a lot of things to pay attention to when you start to bring out those regular expressions. This is because there are a lot of choices that these regular expressions are going to be able to help you out with. One of the nice things about them though is that you aren't just going to bring them out with fixed characters all of the time. you can also use them to help you watch out for a few patterns when needed. A few of the most common patterns that come to play when we use regular expressions in the Python code will include

1. , X, 9, < -- ordinary characters just match themselves exactly. The meta-characters that aren't going to match themselves simply because they have a special meaning include: . ^ $ * ? { [] and more.
2. . (the period)—this is going to match any single except the new line symbol of '\n'
3. 3. \w—this is the lowercase w that is going to match the "word" character. This can be a letter, a digit, or an underbar. Keep in mind that this is the mnemonic and that it is going to match a single word character rather than the whole word.

4. \b—this is the boundary between a non-word and a word.
5. \s—this is going to match a single white space character including the form, form, tab, return, newline, and even space. If you do \S, you are talking about any character that is not a white space.
6. ^ = start, $ = end—these are going to match to the end or the start of your string.
7. \t, \n, \r—these are going to stand for tab, newline, and return
8. \d—this is the decimal digit for all numbers between 0 and 9. Some of the older regex utilities will not support this so be careful when using it
9. \ --this is going to inhibit how special the character is. If you use this if you are uncertain about whether the character has some special meaning or not to ensure that it is treated just like another character.

Of course, these are just a few of the different regular expressions that you will be able to use when you get started in the Python coding language. But they are the ones that are the most important, and the ones that you should learn early on, so make sure to practice them a bit in your codes and on your compiler, to ensure that you are going to get the best results with them possible.

Doing your own queries with regular expressions

In addition to a few of the basic patterns that you will be able to look for in code, like what we showed above, you are able to take some of the regular expressions and use them to complete a search. This search can be done on any input string that is found in your code. There are actually three methods that you are able to use, and as you will see in a moment, there are some definite times when you will decide to use each one.

Each time that you use a program, you may find that you need to re-evaluate which type of query is going to work the way that you want. You will find a use for each one; you just need to make sure that you are pulling them up at the right time. You will discover the different queries that you are able to do when you are on this program when you work with Python and regular expressions.

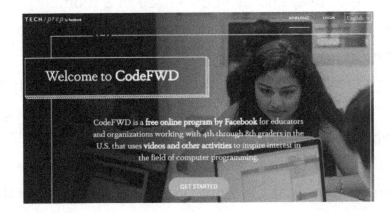

The search method

The first query type that you are able to do with the regular expressions that you have is going to be the search method. This one is a great place to start because you are able to do your query and see if it matches up with any part of the code. The function isn't going to come with restrictions like you will find with some of the others we will look at. If you would like an opportunity to look through the entirety of the string, rather than looking at the beginning, or at the end, then this search method is going to help you get that done.

This search method is going to make it so that a programmer, or a user, is able to go through and look for something, no matter where it may be present inside of the string. Whether the term is in the beginning, at the end, or somewhere in between, you will be able to use the search method to help you find what you want. The syntax that you will need to use in order to bring out the hat search method will include:

```
import re
string = 'apple, orange, mango, orange'
match = re.search(r'orange', string)
print(match.group(0))
```

Before we go any further, it is time to take a moment and add this above syntax into your compiler and see what results you are going to get. For this one in particular, if you did it the proper way, then your output is going to be the word "orange." With this method, you will only see it match up once, regardless of how many times the word of orange ends up showing itself in the string. There could be one orange or twenty oranges; you will get the same output with this one. Once the program has been able to find the first orange, assuming that any string you design is going to have that word in it, then it will stop.

The match method

Now that we have had a chance to work with the search method, it is time to move on to another method that you can focus on. The search method is able to help you in some cases, but there are also going to be times when it is not going to be just right for the code that you want to write out. the match method is going to find the matches to your query, but the location is going to be important. It is only going to pull up the output when your query is right at the beginning of the string. It is going to be responsible for looking out for a specific pattern inside the syntax that you are looking for.

Let's take a look at the example that we did above. You will see that there is going to be a pattern there. This is that the word of orange is going to be between the other words. But when you do the query of re_match, rather than the re_search that we did before, then you aren't going to get a result. This is because the word of orange is not the first one on the list.

Even though you do have the object of orange showing up in the code (and in this case, it is showing up more than once), you are not going to see it show up. This is simply because that word is not the first one in the string. In the case that we are looking at, you find that the word apple is the first one. With this match method, it is only going to do a query of the first word, and if that doesn't match up with what you want, then there is no output.

If you end up having a pattern that is not in the right order when you start out with this, then you won't be able to get the right answers that you want until you change things around. You can change it around while writing the code, but once the code is running, you can't go back through in the middle of the program and make the changes. So, when you are writing out the code, double check that the words end up in the right places along the way.

When you are ready to work with the match method, and you want to see how it works, just take the syntax that we worked on earlier with the search method, but switch out the re_search part with re_match. This is all that you will need to do in order to make this all work the way that you would like.

The findall method

There are also times when you want to be able to find out how many of a particular object is in your string. If you go with the other methods, you will just find out whether the object is the first in the pattern or if there is that object in the string at all. But with the findall method, you will be able to find all of the oranges that are in the string. Using the example above, the findall method would provide you with the output of "orange, orange" since there are two of them present there.

You can have as many of the same object in your string as you would like, or you can pick out any other object as well. If you added ten more oranges in there, the findall method would list out orange ten times. If you wanted to find out how many apples are there, you could use the findall method and in this example, only get apple to show up once.

To see how the findall method will work differently than the search method we discussed before, take a moment and experiment. Bring up your compiler and use the code that we had in the search method. Replace the search part with findall and see what happens.

Then go through and mess around with the list a little bit. Take things away, add more objects, and play around to see what will happen to your output each time that you do this. This is a good way to practice your regular expressions and you can even throw in the match method to learn better how each of these works.

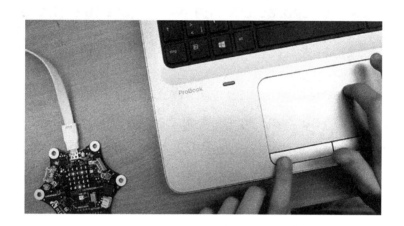

Do I need to use those square brackets?

Before we end this chapter, it is time to take a look at some of the proper coding rules that can make your life easier. As you are writing a lot of the codes that are found in this language, you may find that some square brackets are going to show up in the codes that you are reading. These are going to make it easier to indicate a specific set of characters and will ensure that those are going to be kept apart from the other ones.

A good example is when you would like to write out a statement. You may write it out as [abc], you will then be able to get a match back for a, b, or c. This is going to make it easier because then you are able to get the matches back for them rather than having to do individual searches on each part.

There are other types of characters, such as working with the \w and\s will work with these kinds of square brackets as well, and you want to make sure that these are used. The only exception that comes with this rule is that the dot is just a dot, and you aren't able to go through and match up these, even if you find that they are already in the square brackets from before.

The example that we already went through and did before is a great way to show you what you can do with the regular expressions if you need to add them into your code, and you will need to make sure that you know how to use them to get the results that you would like. There is so much that you are able to do when you work on these regular expressions, and they can come into play, even with some of the more difficult parts of the code that you are trying to work with.

To help you with this a bit more, and to make sure that you have the regular expressions down, it is time to practice a few with your interpreter. Try out some of the examples and mess around with them a bit, seeing how they work and what little adjustments are going to do to the code as a whole.

Conclusion

Thank for making it through to the end of *Python for beginners*, let's hope it was informative and able to provide you with all of the tools you need to achieve your goals whatever they may be.

The next step is to start writing out some of your own codes with the help of the Python coding language. There is so much to love about this coding language, and both beginners and those who have been coding for a long time, and this is why this kind of language has such a following and a community throughout the world.

This guidebook has taken some time to look at the different things that you are able to do when it comes to working with the Python code. From the conditional statements, the loops, working with exceptions, and more, you will soon be on the trail to writing some of your own codes in no time at all.

When you are ready to learn a bit more about working with the Python code and all of the cool things that you are able to do with this kind of coding language, regardless of how much experience you have with technology and coding in the past, make sure to check out this guidebook to help you get started.

Finally, if you found this book useful in any way, a review on Amazon is always appreciated!

CPSIA information can be obtained
at www.ICGtesting.com
Printed in the USA
LVHW081202130221
679242LV00016B/616